Zone Diet

A Thorough Manual On Enhancing Athletic Performance
Through Precise Nutrition, Mastery Of Metabolism, And
Complete Transformation Of The Body

*(Recipes For Optimal Health And Longevity Inspired By
The World's Healthiest Individuals)*

I0089978

DragoBrugger

TABLE OF CONTENT

Blue Zone Green Smoothies

Green smoothies are gaining popularity as a beverage that promotes health. Smoothies that are made with components that are permitted by the blue zone, or "blue zone greens," are becoming more and more popular among those who are health-conscious.

Smoothies that contain solely components approved by the Blue Zone diet, which emphasizes improving health and lifespan, are known as "Blue Zone green smoothies."

Smoothies that are "blue zone green" are a healthy way to get the nutrients your body needs. They are abundant in essential fatty acids, vitamins, minerals, and antioxidants. They are high in fibre and low in calories and sugar, which may help you feel fuller for longer. Alkalizing ingredients included in some blue zone green smoothie ingredients may help maintain a healthy digestive tract and regulate the pH levels in your body.

Smoothies with blue zone green ingredients are also good for losing weight. The mixture of the ingredients aids in boosting your metabolism, which could speed up the process of burning fat.

Of fruits and vegetables through green smoothies. Any combination of fruits and vegetables will do, and it's easy to ensure that each smoothie has a variety of nutrients.

Gain the benefits of a healthy lifestyle by making your blue zone green smoothie right now.

Make your blue zone green smoothie right now if you're looking for a way to improve your health, and make sure you're getting it.

Blue Zone Green Smoothie Benefits

1. Boosts Energy: The nutritious blend of vitamins and minerals in blue zone green smoothies may help improve general health and increase energy levels.

2. Fights Inflammation: Blue zone green smoothies' antioxidants work to reduce oxidative stress and fight inflammation, which may improve overall health and wellness.

3. Enhances Digestion: Blue zone green smoothies' high fibre content aids in better digestion and nutritional absorption by the body.

4. Detoxifies the Body: The powerful detoxifying minerals found in blue zone green smoothies, like spinach, kale, and chlorella, may help the body eliminate pollutants and encourage a healthy lifestyle.

5. Boosts Immunity: Rich in vitamins and minerals, blue zone green smoothies may help to boost the body's innate immunity and reduce the risk of illness.

6. Promotes Skin Health: Blue zone green smoothies' high levels of antioxidants and vitamins may help to improve the skin's look and give it a more vibrant appearance.

7. Improves Mental Health: The inherent nutrients in blue zone green smoothies may help to improve mood, focus, and mental clarity.

8. Encourages Weight Loss: By giving the body muscle gain, blue zone green smoothies may help to support a healthy weight reduction plan.

9. Promotes Heart Health: Blue zone green smoothies may contain abundant antioxidants, vitamins, and minerals.

10. Provides Natural Energy: The body receives natural energy from blue zone green smoothies, which may improve performance and endurance during physical activity.

11. Improves Cognitive Function: Blue zone green smoothies' high levels of antioxidants and vitamins decline.

12. Strengthens Bones: Blue zone green smoothies' high calcium, magnesium, and other

mineral content may help to strengthen bones and reduce the incidence of osteoporosis.

13. Enhances Metabolism: Blue Zone green smoothies' natural ingredients may help to improve the body's metabolism and facilitate more efficient fat burning.

14. Fights Free Radicals: The powerful antioxidants in blue zone green smoothies may help the body combat free radicals and reduce the chance of developing various diseases.

15. Improves Hair Health: Blue Zone green smoothies' vitamins and minerals may help to improve hair's look and give it a more vibrant appearance.

16. Reduces tension: The natural ingredients in blue zone green smoothies have the potential to alleviate tension and foster a sense of calmness.

17. Enhances Brain Health: Blue zone green smoothies' strong antioxidant content may help

to enhance brain function and reduce the chance of cognitive decline.

18. Enhances Vision: The abundance of vitamins and minerals in blue zone green smoothies may help to improve vision and reduce the likelihood of developing eye issues.

The Principles of the Blue Zone Diet

The lifestyles and eating customs of those who live in the world's "Blue Zones" have influenced the development of the Blue Zone Diet. These so-called "Blue Zones" are regions where a sizable portion of the populace survives to be 100 years of age or more and are renowned for their longevity and overall health. Food strongly emphasises several vital elements that support the long life and well-being of these societies.

Using Food as Medicine

In Blue Zones, food is a source of nourishment and a kind of medicine. Whole, unprocessed, nutrient-dense diets are highly valued by the people living in these places. Antioxidants, vitamins, and minerals are all believed to significantly extend life expectancy and prevent chronic diseases.

Plant-Based Diet

The main focus of the Blue Zone Diet is a plant-based diet. Most of the diet in these regions consists of fruits, vegetables, legumes, and whole grains.

These foods are rich in fibre and other nutrients that support good health and help control weight.

The Functions Of Legumes And Grains

Legumes and whole grains are essential parts of the Blue Zone Diet. They are high in fibre, which supports healthy digestion and blood sugar control. Quinoa, barley, and brown rice are popular.

Good Fats and Oils

healthy fats, which are typically obtained from foods like almonds and olive oil. These fats are believed to extend life expectancy and improve overall health since they are associated with a lower risk of heart disease. Olive oil is a key component in many Blue Zone recipes.

Protein Sources

The Blue Zone Diet includes some protein from plant-based foods like fish and lean meats, although it is primarily plant-based. Residents of the Blue Zone frequently consume fish because they live near water sources. However, these forms of animal protein are typically consumed in smaller amounts than in plant-based diets.

Drinks And Hydration

A key element of the Blue Zone Diet is hydration. Although natural fruit juices and herbal teas are frequently used in moderation, water is recommended. Beverages with added sugar and artificial sweeteners are generally shunned due to their perceived health risks.

Mindful Eating Mindful eating is a discipline that is part of the Blue Zone Diet. Residents of the Blue Zone enjoy their food and listen to their bodies' signals of hunger and fullness. Eating relaxed and leisurely facilitates better digestion and reduces the risk of overindulging. In summary, the foundation of the Blue Zone Diet is the notion that nutrition could be a potent tool for extending life and improving overall health. People who embrace plant-based nutrition, whole foods, and mindful eating may benefit from this diet and lead a lifestyle that emulates the positive practices in the world's Blue Zones.

Salmon Baked With Dill And Lemon

Ingredients:

- 4 sprigs fresh dill

- 2 tablespoons olive oil

- 4 salmon fillets

- 2 lemons, sliced

- Salt and pepper to taste

Instructions:

1. Turn the oven on to 375°F, or 190°C.

2. Arrange the salmon fillets on a parchment paper-lined baking pan.

3. Olive oil should be drizzled on the salmon fillets.

4. Add pepper and salt for seasoning.

5. Top each fillet with a slice of lemon and some fresh dill.

6. Bake the salmon for 12 to 15 minutes in a preheated oven or until it is cooked and flake easily with a fork.

7. Warm up the food.

They Are Proteins, Fats, And Carbohydrates.

Fibres are classified as a form of carbohydrate despite being inactive in terms of calories due to their lack of digestion.

The three macronutrients should generally be balanced in meals and snacks.

Several diets suggest varying ratios of the three macronutrients. Still, I like the Zone diet's ratios integrated with the Mediterranean diet and covered here.

While other options can be included in the Zone diet, I will focus on the Mediterranean diet because I believe it to be the most successful.

Remember that a combination of high-fibre proteins, fats, and carbohydrates makes food more filling and delicious [22].

If I'm having a fruit snack, for instance, I feel more satisfied if I add two almonds or some cheese than if I just eat the fruit.

We must avoid even going beyond excessive perfectionism, which would be useless.

Thus, while tracking macronutrients and adhering to a regimen is acceptable, most people do not have to, except athletes, those aiming for particular body composition, and those with medical conditions requiring them to gain or lose fat.

It makes sense that people with certain medical conditions, such as diabetes, cancer, or cardiovascular problems, would benefit from a focused diet and a healthy diet.

However, an unhealthy and inappropriate relationship with food might result from fixating on compulsively measuring macronutrients and obsessively remaining within a set range, especially if you are healthy and at a healthy weight. This could potentially lead to the development of disordered eating tendencies [23].

Since these are highly individualized matters, no definitive guideline can apply to everyone.

Notably, certain individuals could flourish on diets that are low in carbohydrates and high in proteins and fats or low in fat and heavy in carbohydrates.

Nevertheless, macronutrient counting is usually not required, even with these diets.

For instance, choosing low-carb items like non-starchy vegetables, proteins, and fats more frequently than high-glycemic, carbohydrate-rich foods will be sufficient if you feel best on a low-carb diet.

VERY PROCESSED SNACKS

One universal guideline is that cutting back on highly processed foods is crucial to improving your diet.

Certain nutritious foods, such as shelled nuts, canned beans, and frozen fruits and vegetables, have undergone some processing; nevertheless, these are only slight alterations that don't impact the food's nutritional value.

Instead, we should avoid highly processed foods and beverages, including numerous highly processed frozen items with few or no whole food ingredients, canned snacks, mass-produced baked goods, candies, and sugary cereals.

These products typically include substances such as artificial colouring that causes cancer, hydrogenated oils and sweeteners, sugar or even high fructose corn syrup, preservatives and preservatives [24], [25], [26].

A high intake of ultra-processed meals is associated in research with an increased risk of obesity, heart disease, depression, and many other consequences, including cancer [27], [28], and [29].

Conversely, diets deficient in these foods and abundant in complete, nutrient-rich meals have the opposite impact, prolonging life, preventing disease, and enhancing overall physical and mental well-being, which in turn improves outward appearance [30], [31], [32], [33].

Consequently, prioritizing nutrient-rich foods—especially fruits and vegetables- is advisable.

Should you limit your intake of specific foods and beverages for optimum health?

It is best to limit some foods in a balanced diet.

Ultra-processed foods have been linked by decades of scientific research to detrimental health effects, such as an increased risk of illness and early mortality [34], [35], [36], [37], [38], and [39].

It's wise to enhance your health by consuming fewer carbonated beverages, processed meats, and candies.

You don't have to abstain from these foods entirely, though.

Rather, save highly processed meals and beverages for special occasions and prioritize whole, nutrient-dense foods like fruits, vegetables, nuts, seeds, legumes, and seafood.

Goods like candy and ice cream have their place in a balanced, healthful diet, but they shouldn't make up a large portion of your daily caloric intake.

Regretfully, these are high-sugar foods.

BLUE ZONE DIET FUNDAMENTALS IN CHAPTER 2

This chapter explores the fundamental ideas of the Blue Zone diet. This dietary strategy has improved millions of people's quality of life while providing the keys to long life. Gaining from Blue Zone food and starting your path to a longer, better life depends on your ability to comprehend these principles.

2.1 Plant-Based Foods: The Blue Zone Diet's Cornerstone

Plant-based diets are the foundation of Blue Zone diets. People who live in the Blue Zone mostly eat plant-based foods such as fruits, vegetables, legumes, and whole grains. Plants' plethora of vital nutrients, fibre, and antioxidants promote general health and lifespan.

2.1.1 The Star: Vegetables

Vegetables of all hues, tastes, and textures are the main staples of Blue Zone cuisine. Vegetables support immune function, lower the risk of chronic illnesses, and foster vibrant health.

2.1.2 Fruits for Vibrant Sweetness

In Blue Zone diets, fruits are a natural source of sweetness and energy. Packed with natural sugars, vitamins, and minerals, they fulfil your sweet desire healthily, giving you energy and vital nutrients.

2.1.3 Protein and Fiber-Rich Legumes

In the Blue Zone diet, legumes such as beans and lentils are highly valued plant-based protein and fibre sources. In addition to being high in nutrients, they also help with satiety and sensations of fullness.

2.1.4 Complete Grains for Long-Term Energy

In Blue Zone cooking, whole grains like quinoa. They are vital for long life since they offer a variety of minerals, fibre, and steady energy.

2.2 Sources of Lean Protein

Blue Zone diets provide lean protein sources in addition to being mostly plant-based. Depending on the area, this could include fish, tofu, and infrequently tiny portions of lean meat or fowl. Cognitive function is especially abundant in fish.

2.3 Good Fats: Adopting Olive Oil

Olive oil delivers heart-healthy monounsaturated fats and is a staple of Mediterranean Blue Zone diets. Its modest usage as a condiment and in cooking gives food taste and healthy fats.

2.4 Minimal Foods Processed

Avoiding highly processed foods, particularly those heavy in trans fats, artificial additives, and added sugars, is one of the main tenets of Blue Zone diets. The people who live in the Blue Zone preserve their vitality by consuming whole foods with little processing.

2.5 Portion control and mindful eating

Portion control and thoughtful eating are two more essential Blue Zone diet tenets. Eating leisurely, appreciating food, and ceasing when full are common eating habits in the Blue Zone. Better digestion and a greater understanding of hunger and fullness cues are two benefits of this strategy.

2.6 Red Wine's Function (in Moderation)

Moderate red wine consumption is a cultural heritage in various Blue Zone regions, notably Sardinia. In Moderation, red wine is thought to provide some cardiovascular advantages. But it's crucial to comprehend and follow the recommendations for responsible drinking.

Adopting a dietary plan that can improve your health, lengthen your life, and bring the flavours of the Blue Zones to your table begins with an understanding of some basic concepts.

Chapter 4: The Zone Diet's Emphasis on Macronutrients

we gained knowledge about creating balanced meals and configuring our Zone Diet plan. Macronutrients in the Zone Diet in Chapter 4. Knowledge about the functions of proteins, carbs, and fats can enable you to make well-informed decisions and enhance your overall wellness and health.

Proteins' Place in the Zone Diet

Proteins are important to the Zone Diet because they sustain satiety, supply vital nutrients, and help to maintain a balanced metabolic state. The following are some important facets of how proteins function in the Zone Diet:

Protein is recognized to be more satiating than fats or carbohydrates when it comes to controlling appetite and satiety. A sufficient amount of protein at each meal encourages feelings of fullness and pleasure, which lowers the risk of overindulging or unhealthy snacking. Meals high in protein can promote appetite control and hormone regulation related to hunger.

Protein is necessary to form and maintain all tissues, including muscles. Sufficient protein consumption is especially crucial for people who exercise or perform strength training since it promotes the growth and preservation of muscle. The Zone Diet's inclusion of lean protein sources.

Thermic impact of food: This may support attempts to manage weight by causing a modest increase in metabolic rate.

Foods high in protein are frequently high in nutrients, which means they include a variety of vital vitamins, minerals, and amino acids. Lean meats, chicken, fish, eggs, lentils, and tofu are examples of protein sources that you may include in your meals to ensure you're getting the protein you need and other essential elements for good health.

Blood sugar control: Compared to carbs, proteins have less effect on blood sugar levels. Adding protein to your meals can promote. This can promote improved glycemic control, avoid blood sugar spikes, and assist in maintaining stable blood sugar levels.

Balance of macronutrients: According to the Zone Diet, proteins should account for about 30% of each meal, followed by carbohydrates (40%) and healthy fats (30%). This harmonious distribution of macronutrients promotes metabolic balance and steady insulin levels. It enhances energy levels, suppresses appetite, and advances general well-being.

Fish, shellfish, eggs, lentils, and low-fat dairy products when adding proteins to your Zone Diet. When choosing protein sources, it's critical to consider dietary limitations, personal preferences, and demands.

Personalized advice on how much protein is right for you in the Zone Diet can be obtained by speaking with a qualified dietitian or other healthcare provider. It is optimally balanced and promotes enough intake of protein and other nutrients.

Blue Zone Food Recommendations

If you adhere to these guidelines, you will eat more whole, nutrient-dense, and fibre-rich foods—all in a naturally occurring manner.

Plant Angle

Approximately ninety-five per cent of your food is derived from plants or plant products. To no more than one small dish each day. Favourite vegetables: potatoes, carrots, squash, nuts, and seeds. Whole grains are also okay. Even though meat is consumed by people in four out of the five Blue Zones, they do so in different ways. As our advocate, Walter Willett of the Harvard School of Public Health, said, "Meat is like radiation: We don't know the safe level."

Furthermore, research indicates that 30-year-old vegetarian Adventists will likely outlive their meat-eating companions by as many as many years. Numerous health benefits.

When in season, inhabitants in the Blue Zones consume a wide variety of garden vegetables, which they subsequently pickle or dry to enjoy during the off-season. The best long-lasting foods in the Blue Zones diet include leafy greens like spinach, collards, beetroot, turnip tops, carrots, and cilantro. More than 75 different types of edible plants grow like weeds in Indonesia; the phytosterols in red wine are frequently found in weeds. Research has shown that middle-aged individuals who consumed the equivalent of half a cup of cooked green beans every day were half as likely to die in the next four years as those who did not eat any green beans.

Additionally, researchers discovered that individuals consuming a quarter of a pound of fruit daily (about one avocado) had a 60% lower chance of dying over the next four years than those who did not. Many fruits come from plants, all preferred to one avocado. Although we cannot claim that olive oil is the only healthy plant-based oil, it is the most frequently utilized in the Blue Zone diet. Research indicates that consuming olive oil raises good cholesterol and lowers bad cholesterol. In Israel, we discovered that there is approximately a chance of death in half for middle-aged individuals.

How to go about doing it:

Always have your favourite fruits and vegetables on hand. Avoid trying to make yourself eat something you don't enjoy. That might function for a while, but it will fizzle out sooner or later. Try a variety of fruits and vegetables; identify which ones you enjoy and keep your kitchen well-stocked with them. Frozen vegetables will do if you don't have access to fresh, reasonably priced vegetables. (In actuality, because they were flash-frozen during harvest rather than travelling for weeks to your local grocery store's shelves, they frequently contain more nutrients.)

Apply olive oil like a butt. Sauté veggies in olive oil over low heat. Additionally, you can finish boiling or steaming vegetables by brushing them with a small amount of extra virgin olive oil, which you should keep on your table.

Glue up the entire grain. We discovered that oatmeal, barley, broccoli and maize were included in Blue Zone diets worldwide. In these cultures, wheat played a minor role, and the grains they utilized contained less gluten than the modern grains of today.

Whatever vegetables are left in your fridge can be turned into vegetable soup by cutting them, browning them with olive oil and herbs, and adding boiling water to cover them. Simmer until the vegetables are tender, and then season to taste. Freeze what you don't have time to cook in individual or family-sized containers, then serve later in the week or month.

Is The Blue Zone Diet Nutritional?

YeꞒ. The diet was developed by analysing the diets (as well as lifestyles) of the world's healthiest and longest-living populations.

One of the main themes, "plant-based," focuses on getting 95–100% of your diet plant-based. Eating a plant-based diet and depending on foods like tofu and beans for protein is associated with a longer lifespan, according to a study published in the JAMA in August 2019.

Plant-based diets are also linked to a decrease.

Another important trait of the Blue Zones Diet is harahachibu, or eating until you're roughly 80 per cent full. As per the Cleveland Clinic, this diet and method of eating originate from the Okinawawan Diet and is a beneficial strategy to decrease excessive eating, which may lead to weight gain. The Okinawan people also have some of them.

As part of the Blue Zones Diet, wine at 5 is the past tense related to diet. Fascinatingly, there hasn't been a clear-cut, white body of study on drinking wine for a long time. Although the American Heart Association considers moderate alcohol consumption (one glass per day for women and two for men) to be safe, the evidence for the benefits is mixed.

Beginning Blue Zone Diet Guidelines

Exercise Conscientious Consumption

The Okinawan region's Japanese people practice harahachḍbu, or stopping eating when you're 80% full. This trains their attention while they eat. You may realise that sometimes you continue eating not out of hunger but because you want to finish your meal.

Limitations and fosters a positive relationship with your food.

End all activities, such as watching television, so you will be more aware when your hunger disappears.

Reduce Your Dairy Consumption

Seldom do dairy products and milk reach the tables of the Blue Zone populations? Goat dairy products are generally consumed as yoghurt, cheese, and sour milk.

Milk contains lactose, a sugar the human body finds difficult to break down. It is understandable why so many people suffer from lactose intolerance.

Because goat milk contains the enzyme lactase, the body can digest it far more easily. One rule you should follow, therefore, is to keep diapers and wipes, butts, and the like on the low if you are unable to get rid of them completely.

Every Day With A Cup Of Beans

The only food discovered throughout the five regions was beaver.

Fill up on kidney, black, or pinto beans; consume them and ensure they're incorporated into your diet.

Beans include more fibre than other foods, protein, complex carbohydrates (which are difficult to digest), vitamins, and minerals.

They make you feel satisfied for longer and are available in so many variations that it's difficult to become bored.

The next time you go grocery shopping, make sure that beaně are at the top of the list.

95% of your diet should consist of plants.

Nearly all the nourishment that the people in these locations received came from plants, not animals.

Similarly, you can substitute animal products with their plant-based alternatives. Soybeans are a great substitute for, say, almond paste.

People in these regions also practised drying vegetables and fruits to enjoy them longer.

Cut Back on Your Meat Consumption

If animal-based proteins find their way into your meal, the portions should be quite modest, and the frequency of these meals should be seldom and far between. Except for the Adventist communities, every region occasionally consumed meat.

It was frequently consumed during meals and eaten with many vegetables and nutritious grains.

The meat was not consumed in one sitting by them; what was left over was drained and refrigerated for longer.

Prepare Meals and Have Them at Home

People in these neighbourhoods rarely dine except in fast-food restaurants and restaurants.

Cook and eat at home instead of experimenting with restaurant dishes.

For example, some fish, poultry, and meals are renowned for being larger when eaten out than when consumed at home.

Furthermore, you are more likely to adopt a tougher approach with the patients and relatives while you are at home.

Several times a week, eggs are permitted.

A few of the diets that were examined included eggs. They made two to three weekly appearances in the weekly diet of the Adventurers as well as in other places.

You might wish to limit your egg consumption to no more than two times per week because the eggs eaten in these locations are traditionally raised from chickens. Fast-maturing and manufactured eggs may not have the same nutritional value or lower cholesterol levels.

Legume

Legumes, from chickpeas to lentils, are essential to all Blue Zone diets. Packed with fibre and well-known for their heart-healthy benefits, legumes are also an excellent source of. Whether you prefer black-eyed peas or pinto beans, aim for at least a half-cup of legumes daily. Ideal for every meal, legumes complement many vegetable-based meals, as well as salads, soups, and stews.

Dark Leafy Greens: Although any Blue Zone diet includes plenty of leafy greens, dark. Among the healthiest vegetable varieties, dark green leafy vegetables have several vitamins with potent antioxidant qualities, such as vitamins A and C.

Nuts: Like legumes, nuts are a great source of protein, vitamins, and minerals. Additionally, they support heart-healthy, unaffected fats. Some research suggests that incorporating nuts into your diet may help lower your cholesterol levels, which can prevent cardiovascular disease."Nuts are a high-fat food," claims Faller. For example, almonds offer roughly 3.5 grams of fibre in a one-ounce portion. Try breaking a habit from Blue Zone residents and try a handful of almonds, walnuts, pecans, cashews, or Brazil nuts for a healthier snack.

Olivia Oliveira

Olive oil, a mainstay of Blue Zone diets, provides a wealth of health-promoting fatty acids, antioxidants, and chemicals, including olive oil (a chemical known to reduce inflammation). Numerous studies have demonstrated that living without oil can enhance heart health, including monitoring blood pressure and cholesterol levels. Furthermore, emerging research indicates that olive oil may protect against diabetes and Alzheimer's. Choose the most extreme variety of olive oil that is frequently available and use it for cooking, salad dressings, and vegetable dishes. Because olive oil is light and heat-sensitive, store it in a cool, dark area like a kitchen cupboard.

Steel-Cut muesli

The people in Blue Zones frequently select muesli when it comes to entire grains. Steel-cut oats, one of the least processed oats, are a healthier and more satisfying breakfast option. While their cholesterol-lowering power may be their most well-known feature, oats may offer many other health advantages. For example, recent research has determined that antioxidants may protect against diabetes, heart disease, and artery hardening.

Blueberries

For many people who live in Blue Zones, fresh fruit is their preferred dessert. Fruits of almost any kind can be a nutritious dessert or snack, but certain items, like blueberries, may have unfavourable effects. For instance, current research indicates consuming blueberries may contribute to maintaining your bone health as you age. However, the benefits could be far greater. According to another study, blueberries may help prevent heart disease by enhancing blood pressure regulation.

Barley, another whole grain preferred in Blue Zones, may possess chlorophyll-lowering characteristics comparable to muesli. In addition, barley contains essential amino acids and substances that could promote digestion.

PART TWO: BRAKEFAST DIGHTS

Here are three delicious breakfast dishes inspired by Blue Zones and a helpful step-by-step tutorial to help beginners grasp them.

THE MORNING BOWL OF MEDITERRANEAN

Here's a step-by-step guide for making a Mediterranean Morning Bowl that is simple enough for beginners to follow, even if you're not an experienced chef:

Mediterranean Breakfast Bowl: A Snack of Sunflower with the Help of Sea Ingredients:

Greek yoghurt

Freshly blended berries (straw, blue, and raspberries)

Sincerity

Almonds or walnuts

A dash of cinnamon

Staging Station:

Gathering Your Intents:

Start by arranging all of your ingredients on the kitchen counter. Greek yoghurt, fresh blended berries, honey, and a few walnuts or almonds may be required. Remember to bring the cinnamon with you for that final touch!

Choose Your Bowl:

To present your Mediterranean Morning Bowl, pick a pretty bowl. That will be your blank canvas for creating a lovely and delectable breakfast.

Yoghurt Base:

Spoon a generous amount of Greek yoghurt into the bowl's centre. Greek yoghurt is creamy and full of protein, making it a satisfying way to start the day.

Pour in the blended brownies:

Thoroughly wash your fresh blended strawberries and allow them to drip dry. After that, scatter some vivid, colourful strawberries over the yoghurt. Strawberries, blueberries, raspberries, or any other berries you like can be blended and fitted.

A Splash of Honesty:

Pour some honey over your yoghurt and strawberries. The honey imparts a hint of indulgence and natural sweetness.

Nutty Crunch: It's time to include some texture now. Take a small handful of almonds or walnuts, depending on your preference, and roughly chop them. Distribute them evenly throughout the bowl. These nuts now offer healthy fat in addition to a delightful crunch.

Magic with Cinnamon:

Sprinkle some cinnamon on your Mediterranean Morning Bowl to finish it. Cinnamon gives your cake a cosy, somewhat spicy temperature. Like sunshine in a spice jar that is.

Please enjoy the following:

Your Mediterranean Morning Bowl is a delicious breakfast option and a work of art.

Take a spoon and start enjoying every bite. Creamy yoghurt, sweet strawberries, crisp almonds, and fragrant cinnamon combine to create a harmonious blend of tastes and textures.

Rejoice in Gradually:

Always remember to eat thoughtfully and slowly. Indulge in the flavours and allow the contentment of a nutritious and delightful breakfast to permeate your morning.

Clean Up:

After eating breakfast, clean your bowl and cutlery. A clean kitchen equals a happy kitchen!

Here it is - a Mediterranean Morning Bowl that is nutrient-dense and aesthetically pleasing. This breakfast reflects the Mediterranean Blue Zone's healthful eating habits, where people start their days with delicious meals and suitable companionship. Enjoy your gastronomic exploration!

Comprehending The Zone

What is the diet known as The Zone?

Dr. Barry Sears, a writer and biochemist, created the well-known Zone diet in the middle of the 1990s. It's a well-balanced diet that balances the intake of macronutrients (carbs, proteins, and fats) to balance the body's hormone levels. The fundamental idea behind The Zone diet is to keep these macronutrient ratios consistent at each meal: 40% fat, 30% protein, and 40% carbs.

The Zone diet is predicated on maintaining optimal hormonal balance, controlling inflammation, and stabilising blood sugar levels, which may be achieved by consuming the proper ratio of macronutrients. It is thought that people might reach a state known as "the zone," when their bodies function at their best, by sticking to this ratio.

An explanation of the idea and guiding ideas of The Zone

The Zone diet's guiding principles emphasise how macronutrients affect inflammation and hormone control. Dr. Sears claims that the 40:30:30 ratio—carbohydrates, protein, and fat—helps to manage insulin production. The body is thought to burn fat more effectively and sustain steady energy levels throughout the day by controlling insulin levels.

One of the major ideas of The Zone diet is the "block." A block is a measurement unit that calculates how much food is eaten at each meal. A standard block has a set proportion of fat, carbs, and protein. The precise measurements differ according to body size and degree of exercise, but the general objective is to keep the 40:30:30 ratio.

The number of blocks needed daily depends on an individual's goals, activity level, and body composition. Generally, the Zone diet calls for ingesting a specific number of blocks daily, split equally between meals and snacks. The diet seeks to manage inflammation in the body and regulate hormonal responses by meticulously balancing the macronutrients in each block.

Advantages of Dieting in The Zone

Consistent blood sugar: The Zone diet's main goal is to regulate insulin production, which might result in consistent blood sugar levels throughout the day. This could lessen cravings for sweet or high-carb foods and help avoid energy crashes.

Weight management: The Zone diet may help weight loss and maintenance by controlling insulin and encouraging fat burning. Portion control and a balanced macronutrient ratio can help people feel full while consuming fewer calories than they burn, which is crucial for managing their weight.

Better hormonal balance: The Zone diet seeks to maximise hormonal equilibrium by regulating insulin release. Other hormones, including glucagon, which encourages fat breakdown, and eicosanoids, which control inflammation, may also benefit from this.

Decreased inflammation: Heart disease, diabetes, and autoimmune. Fruits, vegetables, and healthy fats are anti-inflammatory foods emphasised in the Zone diet and may help lower inflammation in the body.

Enhanced sports performance: The Zone diet's proponents contend that supplying a constant energy source and aiding in muscle recovery can enhance athletic performance. Nutrition absorption and utilisation may be optimised during exercise with a balanced macronutrient ratio.

Better eating practices: The Zone diet promotes paying attention to portion proportions and emphasising entire, unprocessed foods. This may cause people to eat more healthily and conscientiously, encouraging the development of enduring habits.

Better cardiovascular health: The Zone diet encourages the ingestion of low-glycemic carbs, lean proteins, and healthy fats, all of which can improve cardiovascular health. It may help lessen the risk of heart disease and improve lipid profiles by lowering inflammation and managing insulin levels.

Customisation and flexibility: Although the Zone diet strongly emphasises particular macronutrient ratios, it permits a high degree of dietary freedom. It promotes including a range of fruits, vegetables, whole grains, lean proteins, and healthy fats. Adapting meals to individual tastes and dietary requirements is simpler because of this flexibility.

Long-term sustainability: The Zone diet's emphasis on whole foods and portion restriction and its balanced approach can help ensure long-term sustainability. The Zone diet encourages a balanced, moderate eating plan that can be followed for the long term instead of relying on severe limitations or short-lived diets.

Potential Health Advantages Of A Blue Zone Diet

Research validates several fundamental principles of the Blue Zone diet, which include:

According to, a lower risk of death from heart disease in the general population was linked to a diet higher in plant-based foods.

• A higher diet of whole grains may reduce your risk of pancreatic cancer.

• follows the United States dietary guidelines for whole grains, which recommend no more than three daily servings.

Additionally, a diet high in betaine may lower your chance of developing several cancer forms.

• A Mediterranean-style diet, such as the Blue Zones diet, may also alter your metabolism in ways that could cause you to age more slowly and enhance your cognitive function.

• According to a study, eating more nuts as part of the Blue Zones diet may lower your chance of developing cardiovascular disease.

• A vegetarian and plant-based diet may significantly lower your risk of type 2 diabetes, per an umbrella review published in Nutrients in July 2020. Merely, diets high in processed meat and fish or fish oil-infused vegetable-whitened beef significantly reduced metabolic disease risk.

• sleep longer and better and experience less insomnia.

• Per a study published in Antioxidants in March 2021, phytosterols, or healthful compounds found in plant-based meals, may help prolong life by delaying the onset of age-related diseases, including diabetes and cancer.

Effect of a Blue Zones Diet on Weight Loss

The Blue Zone diet aims to help you live a healthier life rather than assist you in losing weight. However, this healthy eating method may lead to weight loss. According to Dr.Rajagopalal, the diet is based on the principle that whole foods "tendtohavefewer calories thanprocessedforms of carbohydrates, protein, or fats." Therefore, this diet tends to assist people in maintaining a healthier weight because they are not consuming as many calories overall.

Additionally, the Blue Zones diet is high in fibre, a nutrient that supports healthy blood pressure and may aid in weight loss by keeping you full for less calories. Since fibre is an indigestible component of plant-based foods, it fills you up but eventually passes through your digestive system without being fully digested. You might also eat less if you adhere to the 80 per cent diet rule Blue Zones recommends. "When you learn to respect your body's needs and satisfy your hunger, you're eating more in line with them and aren't consuming more calories than you require to be healthy, active, and long-lived," says Cassetty.

Cons and Advantages of the Blue Zones Diet

The Blue Zones diet is a component of an overall lifestyle that emphasises natural movement, pursuing your goals, lowering stress levels, and fostering connections with your community and loved ones. With the Blue Zones diet, you can enjoy all the cancer-fighting, heart-healthy, and other health benefits mentioned above. Specifically, our experts revealed:

• The Blue Zones diet does not require purchasing particular goods or services; instead, it is a farmer's market.

• No laborious counting or measuring is required. You eat according to your hunger level and stop when you are eighty per cent satisfied. You are not required to monitor macros or calendars.

Thus, are there any drawbacks to the Blue Zone diet? Generally speaking, our specialists found no flaws; nonetheless, it might take some time and effort to switch from your existing diet, particularly if you frequently eat quick, convenient items. Cooking may not always be as easy as you think it is. "There might be a significant shift in your eating habits, which requires adjustment," Cassetty explains. You must set aside time to experiment with different cuisines and cooking methods. This application makes it easy to lose weight, tone up, or track your food. "It requires time to educate yourself about the various elements and how to incorporate them into your lifestyle," said the royal family. Instead of completely changing your diet at once, she suggests building on the foods you already eat that are a part of the Blue Zone diet and making one or two other little changes at a time.

How to go about doing it:

+ Find out what three ounces looks like, whether it's three ounces of a larger fish, like prawns or trout, or three ounces of a smaller fish, like oysters or anchovies.

+ Preference mid-range fish such as tuna, salmon, sardines, and anchovies. Avoid predatory seafood such as swordfish, shark, or tuna to imitate a Blue Zone diet. Avoid overfished species such as Chilean sea bass.

+ Steer clear of "farmed" fish because they are usually raised in cramped quarters, necessitating antibiotics, stabilisers, and colouring.

4. DimĖnlʋh Dairy

Reduce the dairy and dairy-related products you consume, such as cheese, cream, and butter.

All Blue Zone diets do not significantly include cow's milk, except that of the Adventurers, which include dairy products and eggs. Dairy products were introduced to the human diet approximately 8,000 to 10,000 years ago, making them a relatively recent addition. Our digestive systems are not designed. We now know that up to 60% of people have some variation in their lactose digestion. This is often an undiagnosed condition.

Arguments against milk frequently centre on its high fat and sugar content. The founder and president of the Physicians Committee for Responsible Milk, Neal Barnard, notes that 49% of the calories in whole milk and almost 70% of the calories in cheese originate from fat, with a large portion of that fat being saturated. Every milk has a sugar content as well. For instance, approximately 55% of the calories in skim milk originate from sugar cane.

While Americans have historically relied on milk for protein and calcium, those in the Blue Zone diet obtain these nutrients from plant-based sources. Gives about the same amount of readily available calcium as one cup of milk.

Small amounts of dairy products made from sheep or goats, particularly full-fat, naturally fermented yoghurt without added sugar, are acceptable a few times a week in a Blue Zone diet. Milk products from goats and sheep figure prominently in the traditional menus of both the Kenyan and the South African blue zones.

We are unsure if people are healthier because of the milk from goats or sheep in the wilderness or if it is simply that people in the Blue Zone go over the same hilly terrain as the wilderness. Generally, most goat milk in the Blue Zone diet is ingested as fermented foods like yoghurt, sour milk, or cheese. Goat milk contains lactose, but it also contains lactase, an enzyme that aids in the body's digestion of lactose.

How to do it:

Try using almond, coconut, or unsulfured soy milk as a dairy alternative. Most taste just as good, if not better, than regular milk and contain just as much protein.

+ Satisfy your sudden desire for cheese by using grass-fed goat or sheep cheese. Try the Sardinia pecorino or Greek feta. Since they are both crisp, you just need a bit to enjoy the food.

VERY PROCESSED SNACKS

One universal guideline is that cutting back on highly processed foods is crucial to improving your diet.

Certain nutritious foods, such as shelled nuts, canned beans, and frozen fruits and vegetables, have undergone some processing; nevertheless, these are only slight alterations that don't impact the food's nutritional value.

Instead, we should avoid highly processed foods and beverages, including numerous highly processed frozen items with few or no whole food ingredients, canned snacks, mass-produced baked goods, candies, and sugary cereals.

These products typically include substances such as artificial colouring that causes cancer, hydrogenated oils and sweeteners, sugar or even high fructose corn syrup, preservatives and preservatives [24], [25], [26].

A high intake of ultra-processed meals is associated in research with an increased risk of obesity, heart disease, depression, and many other consequences, including cancer [27], [28], and [29].

Conversely, diets deficient in these foods and abundant in complete, nutrient-rich meals have the opposite impact, prolonging life, preventing disease, and enhancing overall physical and mental well-being, which in turn improves outward appearance [30], [31], [32], [33].

Consequently, it is advisable to prioritise nutrient-rich foods—especially fruits and vegetables.

Should you limit your intake of specific foods and beverages for optimum health?

It is best to limit some foods in a balanced diet.

Ultra-processed foods have been linked by decades of scientific research to detrimental health effects, such as an increased risk of illness and early mortality [34], [35], [36], [37], [38], and [39].

It's wise to enhance your health by consuming fewer carbonated beverages, processed meats, and candies.

You don't have to abstain from these foods entirely, though.

Rather, save highly processed meals and beverages for special occasions and prioritise whole, nutrient-dense foods like fruits, vegetables, nuts, seeds, legumes, and seafood.

Goods like candy and ice cream have their place in a balanced, healthful intake.

Regretfully, these are high-sugar foods.

MANAGING A HEALTHY DIET THAT WORKS FOR YOU

One of the numerous components of daily existence is food.

Food could be the last thing on your mind after work, errands, family or social obligations, and commuting, among other everyday concerns.

Making food a priority is the first step in eating a better diet.

Spending hours cooking elaborate dinners or preparing meals is unnecessary, but it does need some planning and work, particularly if you lead a hectic lifestyle.

I suggest sensible and successful diets like the Zone, maybe in a Mediterranean variant.

Day Two

• You should eat one-fourth cup of walnuts, half a cup of blueberries, half a cup of oats, and half a cup of nonfat milk for breakfast.

• A snack of one cup of sliced veggies and half a cup of hummus.

• A four-ounce turkey burger for lunch, half a cup of cooked millet, and steaming greens.

• Snack: a quarter cup of granola and a half cup of plain Greek yoghurt

• Tonight's meal consists of a 4-ounce grilled steak, half a cup of brown rice, green beans, and a half cup of roasted red peppers.

Day Three

• One serving of a smoothie for breakfast, consisting of half a cup of nonfat milk, banana, and 1/4 cup of oats.

• Snack: one hard-boiled egg and a slice of fruit

• We'll eat one cup of steamed spinach and one-half grilled chicken for lunch.

• A trail mix snack that is 1/4 of a cup in size.

• We will have half a cup of boiling lentils, one cup of roasted Brussels sprouts, four ounces of roasted salmon, and half a cup of roasted sweet potatoes for dinner.

An explanation of the block calculation process

A key component of the Zone Diet is block counting, which helps you figure out each day. The block calculation process is tailored to meet the unique caloric requirements of each person. Below is a detailed breakdown of the procedure:

How to Calculate Your Daily Energy Needs:

To begin with, you must determine how many calories you require each day. Your level of physical activity, age, weight, and any particular goals you may have (such as maintaining your present weight or decreasing weight) could all play a role in this.

Splitting Up Into Blocks:

Blocks are standardised units that indicate a particular amount of protein, carbs, and fats.

Once you know your daily calorie need, you must divide it into "chunks." A block typically has a fixed amount of calories.

40-30-30 ratio:

The 40-30-30 ratio for proteins, carbs, and fats is part of the Zone Diet. Next, you must determine how many grammes of each macronutrient are required for each block to achieve this ratio. The combined lipids, carbs, and protein blocks should increase your daily energy requirements.

Calculating Food:

It is categorised based on the amount of protein, carbohydrates, and fat in each meal item. To determine how many blocks any food you eat has, use tables or online resources that provide nutritional values.

Organising Meals:

You can arrange your meals to ensure that you get the necessary number of blocks for each macronutrient after you've calculated this. This may entail combining various sources of fats, carbohydrates, and protein to make balanced meals.

Real-world illustration:

Suppose you have determined that you need 2000 calories daily and will consume your calories in 40-30-30 blocks of 100 calories each. Your calorie requirements must be divided into 20 blocks, with 2000 calories per block. To achieve your target ratio, you may wish to arrange your meals to include a specific number of protein, carb, and fat blocks.

Please remember that this is only an example and that the precise computation may differ based on your requirements. It's also a good idea to speak with a dietitian or medical specialist to tailor your diet to your unique requirements.

Blocks of lipids, carbs, and proteins

Blocks are standardised units in the Zone Diet that help manage the ratios of proteins, carbs, and fats and ease meal planning. Each block represents a particular number of calories and a particular percentage of these macronutrients. The general recommendations for the number of grammes of fat, carbohydrates, and protein in a block are listed below:

Proteins:

Roughly seven grams of protein are contained in one protein block.

For instance, if you intend to have three protein blocks at a meal, that comes to about 21 grams.

Glucose:

Nine grams of carbs are found in one carbohydrate block.

Thus, for instance, two carb blocks at a meal would equal roughly 18 grammes of carbohydrates.

Lipids:

There are roughly three grammes of fat in one fat block.

At a meal, if you intend to eat four blocks of fat, that comes to approximately 12 grammes of fat. Therefore, the approximate food composition of a meal consisting of three blocks of protein, two blocks of carbohydrates, and four blocks of fat would be:

21 grammes of protein (3 blocks * 7 grammes each block)

18 grammes of carbohydrates (2 blocks * 9 grams/block)

12 grammes of fat (four blocks * 3 grammes per block)

Hence, the objective is to prepare well-balanced meals and adhere to the 40-30-30 ratio of proteins, carbs, and fats, with the overall blocks meeting your daily calorie requirements.

Please remember that all figures are estimates that could change depending on your demands. To ensure your diet is customised to your unique requirements, speaking with a healthcare provider or dietician is critical.

Section Two

The Blue Zone Diet Program's Fundamentals are plant-based.

Whole, minimally processed meals derived from plants. This indicates that the diet should be centred on fruits, vegetables, legumes, nuts, and seeds, with less or no consumption of animal products like meat, dairy, and eggs. A plant-based diet has various advantages, such as better health results, environmental sustainability, and ethical issues.

Being low in cholesterol and saturated fat and abundant in fibre, vitamins, and minerals is one diet. This may result in better heart health, a decreased chance of developing some cancers, and more effective treatment of long-term conditions, including diabetes and hypertension. It has also been demonstrated that plant-based diets are more environmentally friendly than animal-based diets because they use less land and water in their production.

Focusing on ingesting whole, minimally processed plant foods is essential for a plant-based diet. This can contain a variety of coloured chickpeas and lentils, nuts, and seeds. Plant-based eaters may replace animal goods with plant-based protein sources such as seitan, tofu, and tempeh, while animal items can still be taken in moderation.

good fats

A balanced diet must include healthy fats essential for hormone production, cellular function, and nutrient absorption. But not every fat is made equally. Animal products and processed foods frequently include health issues. Conversely, unsaturated fats, which are present in various foods like avocados, almonds, and seeds, can offer several health advantages.

Two kinds of unsaturated fats that are very. While polyunsaturated fats are necessary fatty acids that the body cannot make on its own, monounsaturated fats can help lower LDL (bad). Demonstrated to lower inflammation and enhance cognitive performance.

Try including nuts, seeds, avocados, and fatty seafood like salmon in your diet to improve your consumption of healthy fats. Given that these meals still contain many calories, eating them in moderation is crucial. This can also be achieved by selecting slimmer meat cuts and low-fat dairy products and removing processed foods.

Trimmed proteins

Building and repairing bodily structures depend on protein, a vital macronutrient. But not every source of protein is made equal. Animal items that are high in protein. Conversely, plant-based protein sources can offer extra nutrients like fibre and antioxidants and are typically lower in fat.

Consider including additional plant-based protein sources in your diet to enhance your consumption of lean proteins. Quinoa and brown rice, nuts and seeds, and soy products like tofu can all be included in this. You can still get your animal protein in moderation, but choose leaner, like sausage and bacon.

Plant-based proteins are a source of protein, but they can also have other health advantages. Legumes, for instance, are high in fibre and may lower cholesterol, but nuts and seeds are strong in good fats and may also help reduce inflammation. You may be certain that you are getting all the nutrients your body requires to perform at its peak by selecting a range of lean protein sources.

complete grains

Because whole grains are high in fibre, vitamins, and minerals, they should be vital to any healthy diet. Whole grains include all of the grain's components, offering extra nutrients and health advantages, removed during processing.

Oats, barley, brown rice, quinoa, and whole wheat are a few whole grains. You can make a lot of different foods with these grains, like salads, soups, and breakfast porridge. It's crucial to carefully read labels when selecting whole grain items because many are labelled as "whole grain" but include a sizable quantity of processed grains.

Try replacing white rice or pasta with whole wheat or brown rice, or select whole grain bread and cereals to enhance your consumption of whole grains. Increase the chance of developing chronic illnesses by increasing the amount of whole grains in your diet.

minimal use of sugar

Consuming too much sugar has been connected. Although the brain and body require some sugar for energy, it's crucial to minimise your meals like soda, candies, and baked goods.

Try consuming fewer processed foods and instead concentrate on whole, minimally processed foods to reduce your sugar intake. All fall under this category. Read food labels carefully and choose packaged goods with minimal or no added sugar.

It's also critical to recognise hidden sugar sources, which can be found in fruit juice, sports drinks, and condiments like ketchup and barbecue sauce. You may enhance your health and lower your chance of developing chronic diseases by cutting back on added sugars and putting more of an emphasis on complete, nutrient-dense foods.

Crimson Fruits And Veggies Zone Red

You are bright and lovely when eating colourful, vibrant, gorgeous fruits and veggies. Enhancing cardiovascular and joint health are the oils found in fish and olive oil. These oils also leave your hair silky and lustrous and your body feeling smooth. Doctors, scientists, and nutrition advisors all advise us to obtain all the nutrients needed to be healthy. Vegetables are a potent source of fuel for the body.

Plants Contain 64 Times More Antioxidants Than Dietary Animals. Antioxidants Aid in the Prevention of Illness and Protect Your Body From Toxins

Generally speaking, veggies contain 65 times more antioxidants than meat. Certain plants have a negative reputation for being low in nutrients. However, this is frequently untrue since while a plant is deficient in one nutrient, it usually contains an abundance of another. Copper, as well as the vitamins B and K, are among the several vital vitamins and minerals found in grapes. In addition to being high in water and fibre, lettuce generally contains phenolic acids, flavonoids, anthocyanins, and vitamins A and C, which are strong in antioxidants. Even fans of Rippley's Believe It or Not may be shocked to learn that iceberg lettuce has more antioxidants than salmon or eggs and that leafy greens like spinach and lettuce contain omega-3 fats. Fish have omega-3 fatty acids, which have antioxidant properties, while plants have a greater variety of antioxidants. These are justifications for regularly incorporating plants—such as fruits, vegetables, and herbs—into your diet.

Fish Are Less Antioxidant Than Plants

Types of Lettuce Variety

Lettuce, including iceberg, romaine, endive, radicchio, Batavia sorrel, and butter leaf mache

Boston Baptist Collard

Swiss Chard spinach with rocket

Kale with loose leaves

escarole, rhubarb, watercress, and oak leaf

Beauty Salads: Nutritious, Satisfying, Slimming, And Prepared ToProceed

One of the greatest dishes for summer is salad. It's one of the best foods all year. Salads are a cuisine that never gets old because there are many ways to prepare them. A salad's base is usually lettuce and many different kinds have different flavours. With only about 100 calories in a medium-to-large head of iceberg lettuce, you may eat as much of this vegetable as you like!

I've never seen a bigger salad; the skinny woman I met ate it.

During a dinner party in a Beverly Hills neighbourhood, we noticed that the party's skinniest woman consumed almost the entire bowl of salad greens herself! It was just lettuce and a mixture of spring greens. As though performing some sort of ritual, she heaped her dish high, drizzled generously with olive oil, squeezed a few lime slices over it, and then threw everything around on her plate. It astounded me that she piled at least three times the usual amount of lettuce on her full-sized dinner plate. I recall thinking before she started eating that there was no way that slender woman could finish that enormous plate of lettuce, yet piece after gigantic bite, she did! The woman was extremely thin, and based on my extensive experience estimating celebrity weight loss for US Weekly and other publications, I estimated that she weighed a mere 100 pounds. Her spouse was a prominent Hollywood film director. I was fascinated by her lack of table etiquette, as she would devour a large salad bite and finish the entire plate while engaging in ceaseless conversation. I was like, whoa! She finished the entire plate. However, as I watched her stroll back to the salad table, she did the same with a second enormous plate full of spring mix lettuce and a dollop of Italian vinaigrette. Observing her finish it the same way, I couldn't help but think, "Wow, you see strange things coming from Hollywood, but this "skinny lettuce lady" is a dinner party mystery playing out right before my eyes." How was she able to accomplish it? Unbelievably, that wasn't all! She returned for a third massive plate of lettuce, finishing it with raspberry vinaigrette, and indeed, she ate every last bite while conversing with the lettuce wedged between her teeth! I just saw the slenderest woman in the room devour at least two pounds of lettuce as if she were competing in a hot dog-eating competition! That was a real-life Hollywood drama, my friend! I never saw such extraordinary eating behaviour, so forget about the evening's entertainment. She would be a great winner in a salad-eating competition.

When I worked in bariatrics with patients who were morbidly obese and had lap bands, I used to assume that if the obese patients had just eaten three plates of lettuce a day rather than attempting to eat regular meals, they could have lost weight. That being said, I still laugh when I think about this woman. But the "thin lettuce lady" showed me something extremely significant about eating patterns through observation. Throughout my twenty years of experience working in bariatric hospitals and weight reduction clinics, I never understood the need to have a personal weight control plan. I am aware that some of my obese patients did not overeat and that the heaviest woman I have ever met ate like a bird—very little at all. She was overweight, though. I discovered that our food habits from childhood persist throughout our lives. The salad was one of the "favourite foods" of the "skinny lettuce lady," who grew up to adore veggies. However, she doesn't enjoy salad; I'll tell you about that incredible fat-burning dish later. The plump woman informed me that she was raised on a diet of cereal and milk in the morning, along with sandwiches—like grilled cheese or peanut butter and jelly sandwiches—sometimes twice a day. That is just too much bread and sugary carbohydrates for anyone to consume. She was obese despite eating very little because none of the foods she was eating were speeding up her slow metabolism, I realised, because all those carbohydrates had destroyed her metabolic set point. She ate processed foods and unhealthy foods, regardless of portion sizes, and even small amounts can cause issues for someone with a severely damaged metabolism. The best foods are those that come directly from nature and are natural. The recipe sections contain information on the finest foods to speed up your metabolism. The "skinny lettuce lady" has discovered which nutritious foods make her feel the happiest, and she lets herself eat as much of these few foods as she likes every day. She told me about a few other things she eats daily, but I only observed her eat salad during the dinner party that night. Meanwhile, the other averagely-built individuals indulged in decadent desserts and fatty treats. "The skinny salad lady" appeared pretty satisfied and was stuffed with lettuce, so she wasn't deprived!

A Comprehensive Of The Blue Zone Diet

Examining the Blue Zone Diet's History and Foundations:

A dietary regimen linked to areas where people live noticeably long and healthy lives is known as the "Blue Zone diet." These areas are referred to as "Blue Zones," and they include locations such as Loma Linda (California, USA), Nicoya (Costa Rica), Ikaria (Greece), and Okinawa (Japan). Dan Buettner, a National Geographic fellow who discovered and investigated these areas, is credited with coining the phrase "Blue Zone".

The Fact is that residents of certain areas have similar dietary and lifestyle practices linked to longer lifespans. Among the fundamental tenets of the Blue Zone diet are:

Plant-Based Foods: The diets of the Blue Zones are primarily plant-based. These inhabitants eat a wide range of fruits, vegetables, whole grains, legumes, and nuts. These foods can support lifespan and excellent health since they are high in fibre, antioxidants, and other nutrients.

Moderation: Regarding their meals, those in the Blue Zone follow portion management and moderation. They eat until they are content but not stuffed, which can assist in avoiding obesity and overindulgence in food.

Restricted Meat Consumption: The Blue Zone diet strongly emphasises restricting meat consumption, particularly red meat, even if it is not fully vegetarian. Rather, they choose lean protein sources like fish and, infrequently, small portions of fowl. This dietary decision is thought to lower the risk of chronic illnesses linked to overindulgence in meat.

Legumes: A Blue Zone diet staple is legumes such as beans, lentils, and chickpeas. They are great providers of fibre, protein, and various vitamins and minerals. Regular legume consumption can provide several health advantages.

The Blue Zone Diet's Scientific Basis and Effect on Longevity:

Scientific studies support the impact of the Blue Zone diet on longevity, which may be explained in multiple ways:

Nutrient Density: The plant-based foods that makeup Blue Zone diets are abundant in vital nutrients and antioxidants that can minimise oxidative stress and inflammation. This may help to delay the ageing process and lower the risk of chronic illnesses.

Fibre Content: Diets high in fibre from whole grains and vegetables support healthy digestion, control blood sugar, and aid in maintaining a healthy weight—all of which are linked to a longer life span.

Good Fats: Nuts and olive oil are two common foods in Blue Zone diets that are rich in.

Social and Lifestyle Factors: Blue Zone communities highly value meaningful work, regular exercise, and a strong sense of purpose. These elements all lower stress and improve mental health, lengthening life.

Dispelling Frequently Held Myths About the Blue Zone Diet:

It's a Strictly Vegetarian Diet: Blue Zone diets are mostly plant-based but may not always follow a vegetarian pattern. Some Blue Zone populations ingest small amounts of animal products, but usually in moderation.

The Blue Zone diet is a collection of principles rather than a strict diet plan, making it a one-size-fits-all approach. It can support longevity and good health while tailored to individual preferences and cultural differences.

It Ensures Longevity: These communities enjoy long, healthy lives partly because of various factors, including the Blue Zone diet. Significant roles are also played by genetics, environment, and lifestyle variables.

In conclusion, the main tenets of the Blue Zone diet include moderation, reduced meat intake, and plant-based foods. Based on scientific evidence, adopting a holistic lifestyle with these dietary concepts may enhance longevity and overall health.

Breakfast in the Blue Zone: Okinawan Sweet Potato Hashed

Ingredients: two medium-sized Okinawan sweet potatoes; one chopped small onion; one diced red bell pepper; two minced garlic cloves
- Two tsp olive oil
Adjust with salt and pepper to taste.
Guidelines:
1. First, prepare the sweet potatoes. Peel and scrub them, then chop them into little cubes. To ensure even cooking, make the cubes about the same size.
2. Saute the Vegetables: Add the red bell pepper and chopped onion. Simmer them for 5 to 7 minutes or until they are tender and the onion is transparent.
3. Add Sweet Potatoes: Fill the skillet with chopped sweet potatoes and minced garlic. To taste, add salt and pepper for seasoning. Make

sure the sweet potatoes are fully coated with the seasonings and olive oil by stirring everything well.

4. Prepare the Hash: Put a lid on the skillet and turn the heat medium. Sweet potatoes should cook for 15 to 20 minutes, stirring occasionally. Use a fork to check the tenderness of the sweet potatoes. Cook for a few more minutes if they are still too firm.

5. Serve: Take the pan off the stove when the sweet potatoes are cooked to your preferred tenderness and a beautiful golden brown colour. If desired, garnish with finely chopped fresh herbs.

6. Have fun: Present your Okinawan Sweet Potato Hash as a delicious and wholesome morning dish. It can be a delicious side dish for different meals as well.

The Blu Zones' Common Dietary Principles

Blue Zones are recognised for their very long lifespans and good health. They share common dietary principles emphasising whole, plant-based foods and mindful eating practices. Their extraordinary longevity and general health are largely attributed to these dietary patterns.

The key dietary principles that are typically followed in blue zones are as follows:

1. A plant-based diet: Plant-based foods, such as fruits, vegetables, legumes (including beans and lentils), whole grains, nuts, and seeds, comprise the bulk of the Blue Zone diet. These foods offer vital vitamins, minerals, fibre, and antioxidants essential for overall health.

2. Diverse Plant Types: Blue Zone diets include various vegetables, frequently cultivated seasonally and locally. Diverse vegetables provide a range of nutrients and health advantages.

3. Moderate Protein Intake: Although plant-based diets are higher in protein, Blue Zone diets contain moderate amounts of lean protein sources. Fish, poultry, and occasionally dairy

products are common protein sources; red meat should only be consumed in moderation.

Blue zone diets, especially monounsaturated fats derived from avocados and olive oil. These lipids have been connected to longevity and heart health.

5. Whole Grains: Oats, brown rice, and whole wheat are examples of whole grains that take precedence over refined grains. They offer essential nutrients and sustained energy.

6. Legumes: Legumes, which include lentils, chickpeas, and beans, are an important source of protein and fibre in Blue Zone diets. They enhance nutritional richness and satisfaction.

7. Seeds and Nuts: Nuts like walnuts and almonds are delicious as snacks or meal additions, as are seeds like chia and flax seeds. These nutrient-dense components offer protein, healthy fats, and a wide range of vitamins and minerals.

8. Minimal Processed Food Consumption: Residents of the Blue Zone generally steer clear of or consume small amounts of processed foods. They hardly ever feature highly processed and sugary items in their diets.

9. Mindful Portion Control: In Blue Zones, mindful eating and portion control are standard practices. Meals are frequently shared, which encourages smaller portion sizes.

10. Hydration: The main beverage options in Blue Zone diets are water and herbal teas. In general, excessive alcohol consumption and sugary beverages should be avoided.

11. Social Dining: In Blue Zones, dining is frequently a shared experience that fosters interpersonal relationships and increases quality time spent with loved ones. Mealtime gatherings with loved ones and friends are treasured cultural customs.

12. Appreciation of Food: Residents in the Blue Zone appreciate and relish their meals. Eating

is regarded as a friendly and pleasurable activity.

13. Intermittent Fasting: Certain Blue Zones include intermittent fasting or calorie restriction practices that are ingrained in their culture and promote longevity.

It's critical to understand that certain foods and dietary patterns may vary within Blue Zones due to regional and cultural differences. Nonetheless, the following diet is primarily plant-based, whole-food-based, and characterised by moderation, mindful eating, and social interaction. These dietary guidelines align with an increasing amount of research demonstrating the benefits of plant-based diets and lifestyle choices for improved longevity and well-being.

The Zone Diet: Chapter 2 - "What to do and what not to do"

You are prepared to proceed to the next phase now that you know the fundamentals, features, and advantages of the Zone Diet over alternative regimens. In this section, I'll discuss which foods belong on your plate and which ones you should try to avoid eating whenever possible. You can still enjoy your diet and hang out with pals once a week, so don't worry. You don't have to worry because of the Zone you may include in your regular diet without losing your sense of taste.

What should I eat?

The Zone Diet allows you to eat a wide variety of foods. In this book, I've gone one step further and given you 75 recipes to get you started and motivated. For you to see how to implement a Zone Diet in your life in a few weeks, I also put them on a two-week meal plan. A summary of some of the foods that are part of the Zone Diet is provided below:

Aubergine

Salmon

Astray

Sea bass almonds, legumes, blueberries with soy cheese Beef fillet

Turkey breast

Breast of chicken

Fillet of pork

Zucchini

Oats with Parsley

broccoli

What to avoid?

Most individuals won't be overly shocked by the items listed above that are allowed on the Zone Diet. Some meals you should be cutting out of your diet now that you're exercising are:

Dairy goods like ice cream, yoghurt, and other items made with whole milk.

It is advised to avoid eating organs like liver or egg yolk, as well as red meat.

Not all fruits and vegetables are the healthiest to eat because some can interfere with your metabolism, such as corn, bananas, raisins, carrots, mangoes and other fruit juices and smoothies.

Steer clear of sugar-filled cereals, white bread, white rice, and other baked products. Whoa! Remember when I said to stay away from potatoes? That's all there is to it.

You have to abstain from all addictive substances, including alcohol, cigarettes, "diet drinks," and other stimulants, to maximise your physical potential.

Achieving the ideal balance between your protein, fat, and carbohydrate intake will help you stay active all day long with less chance of being fatigued. Just as cross-training emphasises whole development, so too should your nutrition strategy.

The list of foods not allowed on the Zone Diet should not deter you. There are a tonne of amazing possibilities available to you. Additionally, I advise you to try the Zone Diet for at least two weeks before making any judgements about it. Most of my customers are taken aback by how simple it is to follow, how delicious the meals are, and—above all—how wonderful it makes them feel to follow it.

Frittata with spinach and mushrooms

Ingredients:

- 1/2 onion, diced
- 2 cloves garlic, minced
- 1/4 cup shredded cheese (optional)
- Salt and pepper to taste
- 6 large eggs
- 1 cup fresh spinach, chopped
- 1 cup mushrooms, sliced

Instructions:

1. Using the sauté option, saute the onions and garlic in the quick electric pressure cooker until aromatic.

2. Cook the spinach and mushrooms together until the spinach wilts and the mushrooms become tender.

3. Pour the egg mixture over the sautéed veggies in the Instant Electric Pressure Cooker.

4. After shutting off the steam, place the cooker on high pressure for 7 minutes.

5. After the cooking time is over, do a fast release after letting the pressure release normally for five minutes.

6. Remove the frittata from the cooker carefully; if you like, top it with shredded cheese.

7. Cut into wedges and reheat.

Cooking Tip: Feel free to add more veggies or herbs to personalise the frittata. When the frittata is still warm, sprinkle the cheese on top so that it melts.

Nutritional Information: This recipe's protein, vitamins, and minerals are well-balanced.

Chapter 2: Advantages Of A Blue Zone Smoothie Made With Plants

1. Better Digestion: The essential dietary fibre in a plant-based Blue Zone smoothie promotes regularity and better digestion.

2. Better Cardiovascular Health: A plant-based blue zone smoothie's fibre, antioxidants, and healthy fats may lower cholesterol, improving cardiovascular health.

3. Enhanced Energy: The smoothie's abundance of nutrients makes it a potentially great energy source to get you through the day.

4. Detoxification: The antioxidants in the blue zone smoothie may aid in the body's removal of toxins and shield it from the damaging effects of free radicals.

5. Weight Loss: The smoothie's high nutritional and low-calorie content may help you feel fuller

for longer and make it easier to maintain a balanced diet.

6. Lower Risk of Disease: The smoothie's antioxidants like diabetes and cancer.

7. Enhanced Immune System: The minerals and vitamins in the smoothie have the potential to strengthen your immune system and keep you in good health.

8. Better Mental Health: The B vitamins in the smoothie may aid in reducing anxiety and improving mental clarity.

9. Better Skin Health: The smoothie's vitamins and antioxidants may help shield your skin from the effects of ageing.

10. Enhanced Metabolism: The smoothie's healthy fats may aid in increasing your metabolism and maintaining an active lifestyle.

11. Better Blood Pressure: The smoothie's fibre and healthy fats may help lower your blood pressure.

12. Better Cognitive Function: The smoothie's omega-3 fatty acids may aid in improving your focus, memory, and concentration.

13. Reduced Inflammation: The smoothie's omega-3 fatty acids and antioxidants may help to lessen the body's inflammatory response.

14. Better Vision: The smoothie's antioxidants may help shield your eyes from damage.

15. Better Bone Health: The smoothie's calcium and magnesium content may contribute to stronger bones.

16. Better Hair Health: The smoothie's vitamins and minerals may help to promote strong, healthy hair development.

17. Better Nail Health: The smoothie's nutrients can help maintain and strengthen your nails.

18. Better Hormone Balance: The healthy fats in the smoothie might assist in keeping your hormones in check and balancing them.

19. Better Sleep: The magnesium in the smoothie can help you get a better night's rest.

20. Better Mood: The B vitamins in the smoothie might help you feel happier and more content.

Quinoa Stir-Fry with Veggies

Components:

One cup of quinoa

Two tsp olive oil

One sliced onion

two minced garlic cloves

One sliced red pepper and one sliced zucchini

one cup florets of broccoli

One cup of snap peas

Two tsp of soy sauce (low sodium)

One-tsp rice vinegar

To taste, add salt and pepper.

Guidelines:

Combine rice vinegar and soy sauce in a small basin.

Combine the soy sauce mixture and cooked quinoa with the vegetables in the pan. Mix thoroughly to blend.

To taste, add salt and pepper for seasoning.

Warm up the food.

SUMMARY AND HEALTH

First, diets that consist primarily of whole, raw, nutrient-dense foods are linked to increased longevity and protection against disease [3, 4, 5, 6, 7, 8]. In contrast, diets that are rich in ultra-processed foods, those that are advertised on TV, are linked to an increase in mortality and a greater risk of diseases like cancer and heart disease.

Are you wondering why aesthetics is subject to the same rules?

Maybe a little fictitious query.

Can someone who is ill be attractive?

It seems impossible for someone ill on the inside to have beauty on the outside.

Understanding that your outward beauty merely reflects your inner beauty is more important than trying to be attractive for the sake of being beautiful. However, this is insufficient because diets heavy in highly processed foods might significantly raise the incidence of depressive symptoms, especially in those who engage in less physical activity [9], [10].

What connection exists between depression and exercise?

They might not want you to know, but research has shown that one of the most effective treatments for depression is exercise.

Extremely dangerous antidepressants are not necessary, and the benefits on appearance will increase your positive mood.

I would like to draw attention to a study [11] that included 156 individuals with Major Depressive Disorder who were identified using conventional clinical procedures.

Three groups of patients were studied: one group underwent aerobic exercise therapy exclusively, another group received antidepressant medication called sertraline, and a third group underwent a combination of the two treatments.

The patient's status in the three treatment groups was evaluated after four months.

The three groups receiving different therapy showed comparable improvements in the participants' quality of life and the percentage of individuals free of depressive symptoms.

However, it was discovered that patients who had improved and/or recovered fully through physical exercise alone and who had continued to exercise on their own had a significantly lower rate of relapse into depression than those who had treated themselves with pills six months after the therapy ended.

It might seem pointless to emphasise how important physical activity is for skin elasticity, muscle tone, and overall look.

Naturally, you're probably not getting enough of some nutrients if your diet consists mostly of ultra-processed foods and beverages like soda, fast food, and sugary grains and consists less of whole foods like fish, nuts, and vegetables. This can have a detrimental effect on your overall health [12] and, consequently, on how you look. Therefore, selecting the appropriate eating pattern from a qualitative and quantitative perspective should come first.

We then look at the significance of mindfulness and exercise.

Thus, having established that "Eating healthy" essentially entails prioritising one's health by providing the body with wholesome food, let's examine how this might be coordinated within individual differences below.

After discussing the significance of eating a balanced diet, let's examine some fundamental nutrition concepts.

HOW TO SAFELY USE YOUR INSTANT ELECTRIC PRESSURE COOKER

To guarantee a seamless and pleasurable cooking experience, it is imperative to use the quick electric pressure cooker securely. The following are some crucial pointers for using the quick electric pressure cooker safely:

Go through the manual: Read the manufacturer's user instructions carefully before using the quick electric pressure cooker. Learn about the appliance's various components, features, and safety measures.

Inspect Valves and Seals: Check for damage or debris on the steam release valve and silicone sealing ring before each usage. Ensure they are clean and placed correctly to avoid steam leaks during cooking.

Add Enough Liquid: Before cooking, always add the necessary liquid, such as broth or water, to the quick electric pressure cooker. There must be enough liquid to create pressure and keep food from burning.

Prevent Overfilling: According to the user manual, do not fill the quick electric pressure cooker above the maximum fill line. Overfilling can result in a dangerous pressure build-up and jam the steam release valve.

Shut Off the Lid Rightly: Before beginning the cooking process, make sure the float valve is down and the lid of the instant electric pressure cooker is firmly closed. To increase the pressure inside the pot, the lid must be closed.

Use Appropriate Ventilation: Make enough room surrounding the quick electric pressure cooker for adequate ventilation, and place it on a firm, heat-resistant surface. Do not use the appliance in small places or beneath cabinets.

Take Care Around Hot Surfaces: The quick electric pressure cooker can get quite hot during and after cooking. Wear oven mitts or silicone mittens when handling the steam release valve and the pot.

Safely Release Pressure: Use the steam release valve or the natural release method (allowing the pressure to drop naturally) to release the pressure after cooking. For the correct approach, refer to the recipe's directions.

Refrain from Opening When Under Pressure: When an instant electric pressure cooker is under pressure, you should never attempt to pry it open. This could be hazardous and lead to the release of hot steam.

Utilise Steam Racks and Trivets: Use steam racks or trivets to raise some foods off the liquid while cooking. This guarantees consistent cooking and keeps food from burning.

Be Aware of Hot Steam: Use caution when opening the steam valve. Keep your hands and face away from the steam discharge region to avoid burns.

You may safely use your instant electric pressure cooker to make tasty and healthful meals while putting everyone's safety in the kitchen first by adhering to these safety precautions. Happy and secure cooking!